MW01644577

# Spirituality for Beginners

A 100 Pages Compact and Effective Guide to Improve Spirituality for Newbies; Achieve a Mindset Full of Wholeness, Positivity, Success, and Calmness Forever, In Less than 48 Hours Part-1

**BY**

**Tom Bhowey**

# Table of Contents

A Brief Introduction Overview on Meditation for Beginners ........ 6
What Is Meditation? ........ 10
Types of Meditation Techniques ........ 20
Why Should I Meditate? ........ 24
Why Music While Meditating Helps ........ 31
Why Use a Meditation Chair? ........ 34
The Scientific Research on Meditation ........ 39
How Science Proves The Effectiveness of Meditation ........ 45
Meditation - The Scientific Method of Self-Study ........ 51
How to Meditate for Beginners ........ 57
Learn How To Meditate Correctly With This Simple 11-Step Guide ........ 63
Meditate to Rid Your Fear of Flying ........ 76
Meditation - Know About Transcendental Meditation ........ 79
The Holosync Solution to Learning Meditation ........ 91

The content within this book has been derived from various sources. Please consult a licensed professional before attempting any techniques outlined in this book.

By reading this document, the reader agrees that under no circumstances is the author responsible for any losses, direct or indirect, which are incurred as a result of the use of information contained within this document, including, but not limited to, — errors, omissions, or inaccuracies.

# A Brief Introduction Overview on Meditation for Beginners

Using simple steps and meditation techniques for beginners, you can learn without having to take time out of your day or out-of-pocket expense to hire an experienced yoga instructor. Most exercises use focused breathing exercises that are easy to learn while listening to instructions on CD right in the privacy of your own home. Once these simple techniques have been mastered, it is easier to move on to advanced meditation techniques as you journey on through meditation.

Focused Breathing. Learning how to focus your breathing is one of the easier meditation techniques for beginners, and this is where anyone would want to begin. Many first-time meditation practitioners feel that they have to learn proper meditation positions for this type of relaxation to be effective, but that is just not the case. The important thing to remember that whether you are sitting in the lotus position, or just sitting in an easy chair, comfort is what you are searching for. Also known as pranayama, the person practicing this exercise begins to breathe at a comfortable rate through the nose, and with the eyes shut. When focused properly, and individual can begin to time each inhalation and exhalation of air over a period of time.

Guided Meditation. Meditation techniques for beginners must also include guided meditation, and this is the most common of the meditation techniques used by those starting out because it is easy and effective. While there are many varieties of style and methods that can be used, the guided portion of this type of meditation is practiced while the individual is listening to a meditation guide. That could be a recording on a CD or other source.

Many times, there will be relaxing music played in the background, or the sounds of nature to help achieve a settled mind while preparing for meditation. The guide speaks to you and sets the tone for meditation, and will go into detail as they describe different scenes and the pattern of breathing you should have. At last, guides will help you to come to a desirable meditative state. That could be sleep or a connection with your inner self.

All of the above meditation techniques for beginners are easy to learn, and can be used to relieve the tensions and stresses of everyday life. They also help to lay a foundation for meditation, and many experts and advanced meditation practitioners freely admit that they continue to use these techniques as they achieve a more relaxed state of mind as well as body.

# What Is Meditation?

You have a way of understanding your own life and the world that opens up new vistas and unplumbed depth. It is called meditation and you should understand something about this amazing innate faculty without having to study for years, join a special group, or learn difficult practices.

There is a depth and breadth and beauty to life which you often may miss. Abraham Maslow coined the term peak experience for that exceptional, joyful, self actualized trans personal special moment. Zen describes an experience known as Satori, which is seeing your essential nature. The Armenian philosopher Gurdjieff talked about how we need to wake up. Yogis speak of a non dualistic awareness known as Samadhi. Nirvana relates to moksha or liberation. All of these wonderful and exalted states actually point back to our essential nature of being. That which you are and remain, when you are not identifying with limited concepts about yourself.

The word meditation has been misunderstood and used incorrectly, especially in the culture of the mass media. Meditation has come to mean everything from contemplating to daydreaming or fantasizing. In Yoga (Ashtanga Yoga) the word for meditation is dhyana and it is not contemplation or imagination. Meditation is a specific practice that quiets the mind, taking us beyond our doubt, anxiety, judgments, in other words, beyond the prison of our mental conditioning. It is a state of consciousness beyond the ordinary waking state. Meditation is a means for understanding and experiencing the center of consciousness within.

Meditation is not a religion, though it plays a part in all the worlds' wisdom traditions and is used to enrich the spiritual experience. Meditation is a science, which means it has defined principles, that there's a specific process which is followed, and it produces results that can be verified.

The practice of meditation is the practice of clearing the mind, allowing it to become relaxed and inwardly focused. Meditation is a state of restful-awareness; your mind is clear, you are fully awake and aware, but your mind is not focused on the external environment or any of the events that are happening around you. You are cultivating an inner state that is one-pointed and still, so that the mind will slip into silence. When this stillness happens, and the mind falls silent and it no longer distracts you, your meditation deepens.

In this 'modern' age, we are not educated in how to look within; all our educational practices are focused on examining the external world. As a result we remain, mostly, unknown to ourselves, strangers to our true nature. Vast reaches of our mind go unknown, the deep reservoir of our unconscious (subconscious) mind remains a mystery and outside of our control. The result is confusion, doubt and disappointment, with these attributes often playing a major role in our lives. It's been said that the whole of the body is in the mind but the mind (the intellect) is not in the whole of the body. It is only through the awareness which arises in meditation that we can really develop control over the mind.

To reach the goal of meditation, which is to go beyond the mind and experience our essential nature, our biggest obstacle is our mind, which stands between us and pure awareness. This is the reason that it is often referred to as the 'monkey mind,' and why the practice of training the mind is compared to that of training a puppy. The mind resists any efforts to control it, because it seems that our mind has a mind of its own. It's the uncontrolled mind that causes us to only experience daydreams, visions and fantasies instead of having the genuine experience of meditation.

The practice of meditation is the practice of stilling and calming yourself, releasing judgment and seeing things as they are. It is a way training the mind so that you won't be caught up in its endless movement and distractions. Meditation is the process of systematically exploring your inner dimensions.

Meditation is a commitment, you are committing yourself to a practice not a ritual or ceremony. Meditation is not about forcing the mind to be quiet (it really can't be done that way); instead it is the process of letting go and discovering the quietness that is always present behind the screen of our internal dialogue. Meditation requires a certain discipline; there is a need for consistency. Me ditation is like learning to play a musical instrument or paint a picture, if you want to reach the level where creativity can flow naturally through you; then you need to practice the techniques until you can let go of them.

Meditation is freedom from the endless noise and distractions inside your head. Meditation allows you to experience what is taking place around you without reacting. Meditation brings you the freedom to experience who you really are, free from all the mental activity, and you begin to experience inner contentment and joy.

This relief and respite from the hectic pace of everyday life is not an escape from the world but the foundation of inner peace. With practice you can begin bringing the attributes of meditation into your everyday activities, which allows you to move more effectively in the world. Applying the principles of meditation to the experiences that happen before you, you can become fully present to them, which gives you time to respond before reacting to them.

Meditation is very beneficial in that way; it exposes your unproductive habits and reflexes instead of acting them out and this leads to inner balance, harmony and freedom.

## Allowing Your Mind To Become Still

Meditation is the way you reconnect with the over arching and underlying essence of your own being. It is a process of uncovering and discovering who you really are in a way that transcends your restricted definitions about who you are and is based on learning how to allow your mind to become still.

## Words You Use Are Only Symbols

It is easy to forget that words are symbols, not the thing itself. When you say a word, communication occurs as someone gets an image and understanding associated with that word, but the word never really possesses the color, flavor, texture, reality and being of the thing the word describes. In meditation you learn to have an open mind, and a quiet mind and this opens up an entirely new way of being, because you begin to be able to perceive things directly without just thinking words about them.

## Contemplation, Concentration, Meditation

Christmas Humphreys used the descriptive phrase, concentration, contemplation, meditation to describe the increasingly deeper process whereby you can still your mind and become more aware of something. Actually, there are fundamental principles of being which can be deeply understood and experienced in no other way, such as infinity, identity and reality.

## Surface View And Unified Understanding

You can adopt a surface view of things and get the general idea, but only through meditation can you touch the deep issues of life that are unchanging, and the questions remain with you until you discover the answers, assuming you're asking the right kind of question. Meditation gives you a basis for understanding that is simply inaccessible in any other way. It opens up a gift you have of knowing things from the inside, where you find the common principle people are describing in their own language and perspective and culture, but when you experience the thing itself, you see the connection that is otherwise missed.

## A Key Idea

Often a mantra or key idea is given as a focus for concentration but quite honestly you may find that this keeps you from really probing the depths of understanding if you aren't able to relate to the ultimate meaning of the word or phrase. You generally begin by directing your attention upward and inward to the center of the forehead, to find a one pointed focus where you can begin to experience a wider and deeper understanding of what Mary Baker Eddy called the incorporeal nature of being, that is now being corroborated by modern subatomic physics.

## Harmony, Clarity, Peace

What is meditation? It is the practice of learning to allow your own thoughts to subside so you can begin to perceive directly the harmony, unity, clarity, joy and peace that are obscured by identifying with and constantly thinking about yourself in a limited, finite way.

# Types of Meditation Techniq ues

Meditation is a practice that has been around for many centuries. The different forms all have well known physical, psychological, and spiritual health benefits. Among these benefits are increased focus, relaxation, and a deeper understanding of yourself and others. But do you know the different types of meditation techniques?

**Traditional Meditation**

A study of the different types of meditation techniques must start with traditional forms of meditation. This form has been around for many centuries. Traditional meditation is what most people think about when they think of meditation. In this form, the meditator focuses in on a mantra, an object, a scripture, image, or a bodily function such as their breathing or heart beat or movement. When the mind wanders, the meditator brings their attention back to the focus of the meditation. This type of meditation takes a long time to master the deeper levels.

## Guided Visualization

Many people have heard of this type of meditation technique. With guided visualization, the focus is on the sound of a voice as it guides you through the meditation. When listening to a recorded guided visualization, this is often accompanied by a soundtrack of some kind, usually either music (particularly the kind that is 60 beats per second or slower), rain or waterfalls, ocean waves, or a combination. The soundtrack adds to the relaxation and the guide helps you get through to deeper levels easier than if you were meditating alone.

## Binaural Meditation

Based on recent scientific discoveries, this is the newest of the different types of meditation techniques. The idea behind binaural meditation is that you listen to sounds being presented to your ears in stereo. Usually, this method is done with a set of headphones so that each ear can receive different signals. The two signals resolve to a frequency that induces a meditative state in the listener. This tec hnique can induce a meditative state that usually only comes with decades of practice using traditional meditation, even for a beginner. The biggest knock on this type of meditation is that it might seem a bit of a "cheat" because very little effort on the part of the meditator is involved. Quite often, you will see the different types of meditation techniques combined in some way. For example, someone doing a guided visualization might also be focusing on their breathing or someone listening to a binaural meditation might also use a mantra. Most forms of meditation, whether it be the more known ones such as yoga, or an old one like tai chi, will fall into one of these main categories. Which of the different types of meditation techniques that you use is not important for most of the benefits, so find a style that you enjoy.

# Why Should I Meditate?

Meditation has been used for thousands and thousands of years. And it certainly has helped millions of people and it still does help many people around the globe. Meditation does not need any help: you can do it on your own, whenever you want to. You don't need any tools nor equipment.

Meditation will help you relax and feel better. Learning how to be aware of the present moment in meditation will keep your mind sharp and help you focus better in other areas of life as well. For example, you may be able to react faster to road conditions, while you are driving or while you are walking in a dangerious environment. Your focus will be on the situation.

To start the meditation you sit in a comfortable position, either you sit on a chair or on the floor. You may also lie down, if you prefer. You can close your eyes or you can keep them open. (I prefer to close them). Then you start to pay attention to your breathing. This is a good way to focus your attention on what is happening right now. Don't try to change your breathing. Just notice how it feels in your lungs, in your throat and in your chest.

If your mind wanders, don't worry and don't feel bad about yourself. Try to notice your thoughts, then let go of them and bring your focus back to the present moment and to your breathing. While you meditate, your whole body relaxes and so does your mind. Anxiety does not so easily pop up while your body is relaxed. It is, however, possible that anxiety presents itself, maybe that you feel certain emo tions, such as anger, impatience, sadness or happiness. Don't try to hold on to or let go of these feelings.

They are part of your experience of the present moment. Keeping your attention on your breathing will help you stay focused and not get lost in the thoughts that your feelings may trigger. Don't ever think that if your mind wanders during meditation, you are doing something wrong. No, that's part of your experience. Meditation is a practice. And part of that practice means being kind and patient with yourself. It also means returning your focus to the present moment.

This process of returning your attention to the present moment can happen over and over again during a meditation session.

Are you ready to give meditation a try? Remember that it takes time to train your brain to focus on the present. So be patient and gentle with yourself. Bear in mind: focus on the present helps reduce stress and anxiety. And that's exactly what you are aiming at, isn't it?

Have you read about the benefits of meditation, and are curious about trying yourself? Perhaps you're wondering what all the fuss is about? If so, read on and we'll take a look at some of the reasons one meditation has become so popular, and how to go about it.

One big reason for meditation's popularity is that it's a great way to relieve stress. Many people live stressful lifestyles these days, and after a busy day of work, it's blissful to get home and finally relax. And meditation provides one of the best ways to relax really deeply.

But how do you do this? Contrary to popular belief, meditation doesn't have to involve twisting yourself into uncomfortable poses for hours on end. In fact, there are many ways to meditate, and there's no one 'right' that will be best for everybody.

The first thing to do is to find a meditation posture that's comfortable for you. You can sit in the lotus position if you really want to, but it's not necessary. Many people meditate by lying down on the bed, or just sitting in a comfortable chair. It helps if your spine is erect and not slouched, but the key thing is that you should be comfortable, so physical aches and pains don't intrude into your session.

As far as the mental aspect of meditation is concerned, some people like to meditate by fixing their thoughts on something specific, such as their breathing, a mantra, or perhaps a flickering candle flame or a meditation recording. It doesn't really matter what the object of your attention is; the point is just to practice keeping your mind focused for a length of time. Doing this is extremely relaxing once you get the hang of it, and gives you a nice break from the chatter of everyday thoughts.

Others might meditate by quieting down the mind completely. Achieving such a state of 'non-thought' can be very challenging for new meditators, but it is doable with practice, and well worth the effort.

Then there are those people who meditate without making any effort to control their thoughts. Instead, they may sit quietly and let thoughts arise as they will, observing them without judgement. If you use this method, try not to get caught up in following your thoughts - just let them pass through your mind and float away, while you remain centred and detached.

You might want to experiment with different methods, to see what works for you. In the beginning you'll properly find that it's hard to keep your thoughts focused or quiet, and your mind will jump around madly. This is normal, and meditation becomes much easier with practice, especially if you use a meditation recording which incorporates brainwave entrainment technologies such as binaural beats.

Such a recording include sounds of specific frequencies which have been proven to help your brain relax and your thoughts slow down. Use of such a track makes meditation much easier for most people, because the brain is getting a kind of 'helping hand'. This can also make meditation more rewarding in the early stages, which is where many people give up because they find their lack of mental focus so frustrating.

# Why Music While Meditating Helps

There are many reasons why music while meditating helps people relax and meditate completely.

First of all, while you do not have to have meditation music, it can help if you have something soothing going on. Many people have found that the music begins to set them into meditation mode because they use the same music all the time, hence, allowing them to relax sooner.

Also, as much as we would like a completely silent area to meditate, exterior sounds often come through. This means that your subconscious is actually checking in on those sounds to check for danger, or an alert signal. By adding music you can actually reduce your subconscious mind's worry over extraneous sounds.

Other people start the music early, because it allows them to sit down and actually meditate. While they finish up chores around the house, or other duties, there body is starting to recognize that it's time to meditate and they find that the actually get the medication done.

Other people feel that music during meditation is the wrong thing to do. If you're curious whether it will help your meditation, you'll have to try a variety of different types of music and sounds. Many types of music are available for download on the Internet, this can allow you a variety until you find the music that works for you, or find out if it actually hinders you.

If your curious as to whether your particular form of meditation can use music as a tool, try it and see if it helps. Then you may need to speak to your meditation supervisor. Often, they may have helpful hints as to what type of music or sounds you should use, or be able to explain to you why you shouldn't use music at all.

# Why Use a Meditation Chair?

Meditation chairs have a lot to offer to the serious meditator. Let's take a look at some of the advantages of meditation chairs, and how they might be able to benefit you.

People meditate for different reasons, and there are lots of different meditation methods. However, most of them involve learning to quieten or focus the mind. Most new meditators struggle with these things, and it can be a challenging process to learn to control that inner 'monkey mind'. And it's even more difficult if you're physically uncomfortable too - in fact, for many people (and certainly most new meditators), it can be downright impossible.

Some beginner meditators make the mistake of thinking they should sit in the lotus position or cross-legged to learn meditation. This isn't the case - go ahead if these postures are comfortable for you, but they're not essential.

If you're one of the many people who doesn't take easily to sitting on the floor to meditate, you can also just lie down on your bed, or sit in an armchair. However, some people find they fall asleep when lying down, and don't have an armchair that provides comfortable support for their back. In this case, a meditation chair can help a lot.

Different types of meditation chairs are available, including tilt chairs with ergonomic designs, meditation cushions (some of which are inflatable) and meditation benches, to name a few. You can also get foldable meditation chairs, which are fully portable and great for anyone who travels or who doesn't have a lot of space.

Chairs and cushions of this type are designed to allow you to sit in a correctly aligned posture. Posture is important in meditation, as poor posture can lead to physical discomfort and make it more difficult to relax. It also impedes energy flow in the body, which is an important consideration if you're meditating as part of an energy work routine.

You might want to try out a few different types of meditation seat, to see which suits you best. You might find that sitting in such a chair feels a bit strange, especially if you're accustomed to slouching on the sofa. These chairs are designed to stop you your slumping your back and shoulders, and it might feel like it takes some effort to maintain an optimal position. You should find however, that mainta ining such a posture is easier in a meditation chair than it would be on the floor or a squishy armchair, and once you get used to it, you'll discover how this good alignment helps your concentration and mental clarity as well as keeping your body comfortable.

You might want to look for an adjustable meditation chair, especially if you're taller or shorter than average, are overweight or have any mobility issues. These chairs may cost a bit more, but are a good investment if you want to make the most of your meditation practice. If you attend a meditation class with a teacher or know any experienced meditators, it's also worth asking their opinions about the chairs you're considering, to help make your choice.

A meditation chair isn't essential for effective meditation, but it can help a lot, especially if you find sitting on the floor difficult or are prone to falling asleep when lying down. Meditation isn't supposed to be hard or painful, so don't make things more difficult than they need to be by forcing yourself to sit in an uncomfortable position when there are alternatives available!

# The Scientific Research on Meditation

Meditation is a practice first initiated by the Buddhists and has now successfully spread all over the world. Later on many scientific researches were conducted on the techniques of meditation after which it became evident that it truly does have a great beneficial effect on the health of a person. But before you go on to understand how and why meditation works it's important that you first understand the process of meditation. Especially for all those people who haven't yet given it a try and often wonder if it can really work, understanding this process will really help them comprehend the process of meditation.

Meditation is based on two major steps. The first step involves the development of both physical and mental calmness. Once that stage is achieved you go on to the next step of meditation which involves heightening the level of sensitivity, awareness, and observation. The trick to enjoying the full benefits of meditation is to be able to attain both these steps and levels at the same time. For beginners its best to take one step at a time and ensure that you have a full grip on enabling yourself to achieve physical and mental calmness before you move on to the next stage. It is the ability to emphasize on the present moment without being bothered by any of the past or surrounding distractions that makes meditation successful.

Looking at someone meditate may seem to others as a piece of cake. But the reality is that achieving those true states required in meditation is not easy. It requires a lot of hard work and practice. But it has been scientifically proven that a person who regularly indulges in meditation has the ability to bring forth positive changes to his or her brain. The concept of meditation is pretty much based on the facts that when you see a sad movie you instantly feel sad and even hours after watching that movie the effects still linger on. Whereas when you see a comedy movie you laugh out loud which helps you get into a happy mood and hours after watching the movie you feel fresh.

These days scientists are struggling to come up with a mechanism that will help people in meditation by enabling them to avoid all that hard work. By injecting electrodes in the human brain, scientists have been able to achieve that same state of mind that meditation helps a person achieve. It was the neuroscientists of the Massachusetts University of Technology and Stanford University that first established this theory of meditation when they successfully induced a wave pattern in the brains of mice that was similar to the one meditation brings forth.

The benefits of meditation are far more than you can imagine. By gaining more experience in the practice and by mastering the art you can enjoy some great positive effects to your brain by giving yourself an hour or two daily for meditation. Within a few months of practicing meditation you will feel that you have greatly changed and improved your health.

Scientific research of brainwaves shows that meditation can really improve health and well being of a person. Neuroscientists found that people who meditate can shift the brain activity to different areas of the brain. This kind of shift decreases the effects of stress and anxiety. That's why these people are happier and calmer than before.

There an experiment was conducted with two groups of people from high-tech industry. One group was instructed to meditate for a few minutes a day for eight weeks. Another control group was left alone without such instruction. The brainwaves of all people who participated in the experiment were recorded three times. First time it was recorded in the beginning of experiment. Second time it was recorded at the end of the experiment. The third time brainwaves were recorded four month after the experiment. These measurements showed that people who have meditated for eight weeks have brainwave patterns that correspond to calmer and happier state.

Other studies have shown that meditation improves not only psychological state of a person but also physiological condition. For example regular meditation can help to reverse heart disease. Meditation can release pain and improve immune system. Here is a specific example that was published in journal Stroke. African-American people have twice as much risk to die from cardiovascular disease than white people.

So the experiment was conducted with 60 African-Americans who had atherosclerosis. They practiced meditation for six to nine months. Those who meditated showed significant decrease in the hardening of their arteries. Whereas another control group of people who did not meditate showed increase in hardening the arteries. That study showed that meditation could potentially bring decrease of risk of heart attack by 11 percent and decrease of strokes by 15 percent.

# How Science Proves The Effectiveness of Meditation

When people hear the term meditation, they instantly connect it with archaic spiritual and pseudoscientific practices,but the truth remains that not only meditation has immense scientifically proved benefits but it also based on the principles of science. Contrary to the common belief that meditation is all about sitting still, there are actually numerous ways to meditate even on the go.

A lot of the methods involve meditation in some sort of motion, but does this really have a scientific base or are we just romanticizing a concept based on more of a placebo effect? While some continue to negate the link, here's taking a look at how science proves the healing power of meditation.

Effect of Meditation on Brain Waves, and consequently on the state of the mind- It is already established that brain uses electromagnetic waves to function. There are different types of brain waves- the Beta Wave that are responsible for logical thinking, awareness, the Alpha Wave concerned with meditation, relaxation, the Theta wave concerned with an out-of-the body experience or daydreaming. A study testing the efficacy of Sahaja Yoga confirmed that during the test phase the meditators experienced pre-dominant Alpha waves.

Meditation Increases Concentration Span- Well this is actually no rocket science. In today's era where the maximum attention span is of 6 seconds, it is very difficult to concentrate on anything for long. A study published in PLOS Biology suggests that three months of consistent meditation can train the brain to increase the attention span. The director of the Center for Mind and Brain at the California University spoke in context of the study and called it neuroscience evidence' that changes the working of the brain through meditation.

Meditation can help lower blood pressure- In a study conducted on 200 heart patients, it was found that patients who meditated on a regular scale had over the time shown a decrease in the blood pressure. It is to be noted that all of these patients had heart conditions. Those who meditated were also disease free comparatively than those who did not meditate. It was also found that meditation helps to reduce the systolic blood pressure by an average of five millimeters of mercury.

Meditation increases the reasoning power- When a person meditates, their minds are in a state of calm. The basic principle of meditation is to induce calm by getting rid of the random thoughts that charge throughout the mind, and one which makes reasoning difficult by clouding it with other unrelated thoughts. A research conducted at UCLA using MRI showed that among the group of subjects, certain areas of the brain of those who meditated regularly were larger. Basically these areas were the ones associated with emotions, which is why meditation is also recommended to those with emotionally triggered disorders. Since meditation gives the power to control the emotions, it indirectly also makes a person's ability to reason out better.

Meditation builds up a healthier brain- Ask someone who meditates on a regular basis and have been doing so for years, they will tell you how they do not need a lot of sleep or tons of caffeine to charge their minds and bodies. Those who meditate condition their brains over a period of time to become healthier. Getting rid of negative thoughts, improving concentration power and attention span, and the ability to think and reason out better are all important requirements of a healthy brain and hence a healthy body. And studies conducted on a group of meditators proved that meditation does indeed help in improving the overall health of the brain.

Meditation reduces anxiety, stress, and depression- Probably a no-brainer since meditation is highly recommended for anyone going through or has stress and depression issues. According to

a study published in Psychosomatic Medicine in 2009, the effects of meditation on stress and depression was calculated and it was established that meditation does indeed help to both reduce the level of stress and anxiety, and help with depression while at the same time it empowers the meditator to fight against these, thus working as a preventive measure as well.

The concept is still in its infancy and every day a number of studies and researches are being conducted to understand the link better and to scientifically quantify or deny meditation which has a therapeutic effect. Having said that, meditation does indeed work wonders for our overall mental and physical health, from attaining peace of mind to control over emotions.

While we are yet to prove the concept of meditation through scientific laws and formulas, it is safe to say that the benefits of meditation have already been established as per studies and experiments. For anyone looking to overcome emotional problems and mental disorders, meditation does make it a lot easier, and this is why even doctors strongly recommend this.

# Meditation - The Scientific Method of Self-Study

Metaphysics, Meditation, and spiritual matters in general tend to be plagued by sloppy thinking. While we do want to be open to new possibilities (this is at the core of properly applied science), we want to have a structured approach to our practice, whatever it may be.

What follows is the modified scientific method for the study of the self.

- ✓ Recognizing a Problem
- ✓ Perform some research/Form a hypothesis
- ✓ Design exercises, or play with exercises you found
- ✓ Pay close attention to the subjective results you get (use a journal)

- ✓ Form working conclusions and continue experimentation

Step 1 does not really require a problem, just something you would like to change or improve. Mindfulness is your best friend here. If you want to work on the self or explore the self, it helps to have an awareness of the components of self first. If you have never taken the time to pay close attention to your 5 primary senses or your thinking senses of internal pictures or internal sounds, now is the time to start.

Step 2 suggests that you research the area a bit before formulating your own hypothesis. You don't have to make your hypothesis based on this research, but it helps to know what other people who have worked the field have come up with thus far.

Step 3 encourages us to really get to work. This is where we allot time for meditation or other exercises and follow through. This is where we actually run the experiment, and the experimentation never truly ends. It might change direction, but it will continue.

Step 4 reminds us to track our results. Write down detailed descriptions of your subjective experience as you go. This gives points of reference for the changes you have experienced. When looking through the eyes of the new you, it might not be easy to see how much different you are now from the way you used to be.

Step 5 allows us to put working principles in place to help us continue with further experimentation. Keep in mind, these are just working theories; they are subject to change and improvement.

To illustrate, allow me to share an example from my own life. Several years back, when I was still in the Army, I started meditating every day before I went to work. As I continued practicing, the meditations grew deeper, and it made the early part of the day more pleasant at work. I noticed, however, that I wasn't really developing the ability to deal with my day-to-day challenges in a 'meditative' way (step 1).

It was like a peak experience that would wear off. I read through some of the meditation books I had at the time, but did not find anything that really applied to what I was experiencing (step 2). I figured if I could find a way to practice in the morning or throughout the day, I could experience more freedom when challenges come up. So I started playing with quick methods of meditating, and short meditative exercises (step 3). I wasn't very good at keeping a journal at the time, but I did measure my satisfaction with the day, as well as individual experiences with and without applying the techniques (step 4). Based off this, I continued to test and practice these methods to this day. A vastly simplified version of my results would be "When I'm in a good space, I get better results. When I'm in a bad space, I get worse results."

This is only one example, but you can apply this method virtually anywhere in your life. When you do, you will get powerful, measurable results!

# How to Meditate for Beginners

Meditation has been around for thousands of years, early Indian scriptures known as "tantras" first made references of meditation techniques over 5,000 years ago. Buddha promoted meditation far and wide across the Asian continent around 500 B.C which was adopted and further customized among different cultures, religions, and ethnic groups.

As early as the 1920's and 1930's Edgar Cayce promoted meditation and wrote...

"These, as we find, are slow, yet sure, if there will be kept, not only the corrections made occasionally, once a month or such, might be the more often but the meditation; and in the meditation, don't meditate upon, but listen to the voice within. For prayer is supplication for direction, for understanding. Meditation is listening to the Divine within. (Cayce Reading 1861-19)"

But it wasn't really until the 1960's and 1970's when meditation began to make inroads into western society when many professors and researchers began conducting studies and learning how to meditate to test the effects of meditation and its multitude of benefits. This research has proven that meditation provides enormous positive effects on an individuals overall health and spiritual wellbeing.

So what steps must one take to learn how to meditate for beginners? In its simplest form meditation is stilling our mind and body by focusing on our god spirit within instead of the world around us. Studies have shown a minimum of 11 minutes of daily meditation is needed to get the best results including a sense of peace which carries over into your waking life.

For those who are interested in learning how to meditate, there are a few forms of meditation one could pursue. They may vary based on physical motions such as yoga prana breathing techniques, or mental techniques such as meditation which involves clearing your mind of all thoughts, feelings, and emotions usually by focusing on a mantra or affirmation. Blanking your mind may sound easy to do but it's much harder than you think and not recommended when learning how to meditate for beginners.

According to Edgar Cayce clearing your thoughts is not even necessary as the mind is "a constructive force and allows for the closest attunement possible if used in the right way." In other words, through visualizations such as seeing what you desire in your mind, you can utilize the law of attraction and draw what you desire in life.

Meditation provides three levels of benefits. Physically we can relax; mentally our negative thoughts and ego and become quiet and focused; and spiritually we can feel energized, loved, and able to deal with other people and events in a much more positive way.

When adopting a meditation regime its best to place yourself on a daily ritual so you won't forget or be distracted by life daily activities that you will forget. Remember just like if you forget to eat, your body can become fatigued, so too with meditation, if you forget then your spiritual body can become run down and you start to lose touch with your connection with god.

The best place to meditate is a place where you can find quiet without distractions such as bedroom, bathroom, or even car provided you are not driving while meditating. At this point you may want to slow down your breathing and become aware of each breath as you begin to relax. Then bring your awareness to whatever it is on your mind and ask the universe to show you the answers you seek.

You may even want to try tools to assist you such as a guided meditation audio recording. Many of these can be purchase from many online sources such as eBay or Amazon, or you can download them for free off YouTube using a wonderful tool known as snipmp3.com.

Guided meditation audio tracks are great when learning how to breathe properly and how to focus your mind on whatever you desire. They are also wonderful for people who have trouble visualizing in their mind and those not sensitive to chakras or chi energy fields.

Another great tool is the Neo Meditation cube which brings chi energy into your body. The cube is based on sacred geometries and channels consciousness energy into thought manifestation. You could consider them reality generators as they help users bring their desires into fruition using the power of the god force within. So whatever method you choose be confident in your ability to create your own reality and walk with full faith in the divine path god has ordained for all of us.

# Learn How To Meditate Correctly With This Simple 11-Step Guide

Once you have learned how to meditate properly and started progressing in your practice, you will effectively benefit from a healthier body, with improved energy levels, immune system and longevity; a sharper mind, with increased mental strength, focus and memory retention/recall, as well as emotional well-being, with reduced stress, worry, anxiety and/or depression and enhanced self-confidence, optimism and vitality.

On a mystical, more profound level, meditation also known as "the Fundamental Practice" confers the return to one's pure nature and mind, free from the emotional upheaval of suffering through the defilements of hatred, anger, delusion and other impure, mundane imperfections of the mind. As the mind goes passive, clear and serene, just like a mirror, with no thoughts of any nature (good or evil), meditation will unfold naturally, allowing you to get in touch with your own self's nature through wisdom, liberating all that energy trapped by worldly illusions and bestowing upon you inner peace and a deep, intense kind of healing.

Below is an easy, simple and useful 10-step guide to help you learn how to meditate correctly.

**1. Proper Posture**

For meditation to come about, it is vitally important to hold your back upright, with your head up, while cross-legged on the floor (full-lotus) or sitting on a chair. Since the body and mind are intimately connected, a proper and well-balanced posture will reflect itself upon your mind. Failing to sit up with your spine straight and shoulders back, will make your thoughts drift away and you will be tempted to follow them.

One way to help you sit properly erect and purify your mind is to envision your head touching the sky.

## 2. A Quiet Place of Your Own

You should advisedly find a well-ventilated, uncluttered and tranquil place where you can sit undisturbed for anywhere between 20 minutes to an hour or more on a regular basis. Be sure to let personal comfort guide you in the beginning, setting up a schedule you can live with and stick to. It would be ideal if you could create a special little place where meditation can naturally unfold. Even better, you can create an altar or a shrine that you can face during meditation. Here you can place candles or other natural objects that strike a chord with you and have a calming and relaxing effect on you, such as stones, crystals, flowers or seashells.

## 3. Eyes ( Half-Open or Closed)

While most people associate the meditation practice with keeping the eyes closed (as in Vipassana meditation) and mentally drawing the eyes toward the third eye, the choice of keeping your eyes half open or closed while meditating is entirely yours, as there no right or wrong way in terms of what to do with the eyes (in fact this varies among different meditational methods and even teachers). While some argue that thoughts tend to drift when keeping the eyes closed, others prefer closed eyes during meditation, precisely because this helps them focus better. On the other hand, some recommend keeping your eyes half or partly open and letting your gaze gently downward and soft, as this method allows you to be effectively more present. Overall, you should advisedly experiment with both half-open and closed eyes methods and see what works for you. For your advancement, it is crucial to relax the muscles around the eyes and choose the method you are most comfortable with.

**4. Focus**

Meditation is a proven wake-up call that fine-tunes your body, mind and spirit to realize the true essence of life. In ordinary life, focus equates to concentration where we use our mind as a focused beam of light to achieve our mundane goals. In meditation on the other hand, focus has different connotations and using our tortured, disorganized minds immersed in turmoil is not helpful. When practising meditation, focus means paying careful attention to whatever you place at the core of awareness. When you focus your thoughts and practice in complete absorption, oblivious to your surroundings, you become empowered in many different ways. In Ch'an (or Zen) tradition, the breath is used as focus, because it's regarded as a natural door connecting outside and inside. Relaxed and sustained focus of this kind effortlessly becomes meditation.

## 5. Breathing

Paying close attention to your natural breathing is an important part of learning how to meditate. The abdomen expands and relaxes as you inhale and contracts as you exhale. Observe your breathing, but refrain from regulating it because it's paramount to come natural. As your focus strengthens, your breathing starts to slow down and deepen, becoming quite subtle and increasingly finer. You will effortlessly begin to relax once residual tension has faded away and will experience a state of well-being, tranquility and peacefulness. You should devote at least a couple of minutes per day to this breathing relaxation practice.

## 6. Counting your breaths

In case you are having trouble relaxing so that calm can ensue, you may try the ancient meditation practice of mentally counting your breaths - "one" as you breathe in, "two" as you breathe out, "three" as you breathe in again and "four" as you breathe out; then go back to "one". Whenever your thoughts tend to wander, breath counting can help you settle and clear your mind. Returning to "one" allows you to anchor yourself in the present moment and focus your awareness on your breathing.

## 7. Thoughts

Meditation takes place in the absence of thoughts; when you notice thoughts hovering over your mind, you should gently let them disappear on their own by staying focused on your breath. Trying to forcefully stop thoughts will only make you feel more unsettled and anxious. The mind that doesn't dwell on anything is known in the Buddhist tradition as the "original nature" or "true mind". One way to let thoughts go naturally is to imagine they are unwelcome visitors that you politely ask to leave. At no time should anything feel uncomfortable or forced; instead, it should all happen free of any concern or worry on your part.

**8. Silence**

You may try practising with the aid of meditation music, but the best results are achieved when sitting in complete silence, because as you progress in your meditation practice, the outer and inner silence come together, giving way to a profound kind of healing. Sitting erect in pure silence allows the mind to properly settle and to grow quiet and calm.

**9. Emotions**

When you feel overwhelmed by powerful emotions such as fear, anger, shame and frustration, which are bound to give way to unsettling stories in your mind, you may find sitting down to meditate quite difficult. The best way to deal with such strong emotions when learning how to meditate is by re-focusing on your bodily sensations that reflect these emotions. Different emotional states have been scientifically proven to be intimately connected to a wide array of physiological changes or body feelings, ranging from the racing pulse that results from fear or anger (felt in the upper chest area) and sweaty palms when we are nervous of anxious, to the glorious feeling of happiness, felt from head to toe. By directing all your attention to your bodily sensations, you are acknowledging your emotions without being caught up in the stories arising from them, which in turn enables your mind to put them behind you.

### 10. Duration

Advisedly start by sitting anywhere from a couple of minutes to 10 minutes or for as long as you feel completely comfortable, whenever you happen to think of meditation. Do not force yourself to sit for longer periods as you learn how to meditate if you experience any discomfort or restlessness after some time. You can gradually increase the duration of your meditation to 20-25 minutes, which allows you to stabilize your mind without causing a lot of stress on your physical body, and in time, to even an hour or more per day. The most important thing is to do what feels right and especially comfortable for you.

## 11. Delight

Equally important is to take great delight in practising meditation because enjoyment holds a powerful significance over the outcome of your entire efforts. In keeping with the Kalama Sutra, do not do something because you have been told to do so, but instead find out what works for you. Don't put pressure onto yourself - just be kind to yourself and let meditation unfold naturally, as it should. Take it slowly as you learn how to meditate, sitting a few minutes each day, with a hint of smile on your face. As you advance in your practice, you are required to sit motionless for longer periods of time and then you may need to make some adjustments in the way you sit.

The art of meditation is as old as the mountains and as profound as the deepest ocean. Every religion and every spiritual practice preaches meditation in some form or the other. It may be through chanting the scared 'Om' or praying five times a day, such as the whole act of participating in 'namaaz'. Meditation is the act of being one with your body with your every breathing moment.

Meditation is an exercise, which allows your mind to be free of scattered thoughts. A free mind guides the practitioner to his inner peace and ultimate realization of bliss. Just as our body requires physical activity to be fit, meditation is a mental activity for the mind to function in tandem with the body. It is more than attaining a physical posture, closing the eyes, and taking breath control.

**Find a Place**

Find a place that is calm, quiet, and totally noiseless. Sit down with your legs crossed and get familiar with the ambiance. Rest your hands on your lap and try to relax. Get comfortable in the position. Use a chair if you can't sit in the cross-legged position for long. It's not necessary to attain a lotus position for meditation, in the beginning. It's more important to focus on the art and its act.

**Being There**

If you are a first timer, your mind will wander different planes. Your thoughts will distract your every breathing moment, and your mind will make you think of everything you should not. Don't be discouraged. It happens to everyone. The point here, is to still push yourself to retain the position for at least 15 minutes. Bring your mind back on track, every time it tries to scoot off somewhere. Within a week of this drill, you will feel much more calmer, and you will be able to focus better. Meditation will eventually give you the power to hold your mind by a tight leash. It's an exhilarating boon, trust me on this one!

**Breath Control**

Begin with closing your eyes gently and take a few slow, pronounced deep breaths. Inhale from your nose and exhale from your mouth, for the first 10 breaths. Then inhale and exhale from your nose. Feel the cool breath on your upper lip and feel and warm breath leaving your body. Never force breathing, as it will keep disturbing your natural tempo. The initial breathing will seem shallow. As time progresses, you will automatically allow more air to fill your lungs, making your breaths deeper and deeper. Take long slow breath, when you reach this point and continue breathing deeply.

# Meditate to Rid Your Fear of Flying

Meditation can be one of the best ways to help you rid of your fear of flying or at least help you control it. Fear of flying is one of the most common fears among people. The fear of flying can become such a problem that sometimes it can give you sleepless nights before boarding an airplane; it can give you panic attacks among other stresses that can end up in your body as some form of disease. Meditation relaxes the body and helps reduce stress by putting your body and mind at ease. It has helped so many that it has become a popular method to help those with the fear of flying and it comes with secondary benefits; it helps people handle other concerns in their lives.

The thought of Meditation sometimes stops people from getting rid of their fears. The meditation is an easy and once you learn the process it can be enjoyable; meditation is done by many and are enjoying the benefits. There are many ways to learn about getting rid of your flying fears; listening to CDs', reading online or store bought books, searching online about what people are writing about this topic. It is endless the available information. Listening to a CD might be easier as it can be carried with you everywhere you go and you can listen while driving your car, at home, at work, even before boarding an airplane and during the flight. The meditation courses will help you get rid of your flying fears but they will also teach you how to deal with other fears you might be having; it will help eliminate your anxieties about flying but it will be useful in other areas of apprehension you might have in your life.

The meditation CDs' are being made available by some airline companies; they are beginning to provide them to passengers to help them relax aboard the plane. They have notice this benefit cuts both ways by serving themselves and the more relaxed passenger will be more willing to travel more often. The airlines have become very creative in the types of meditation CDs' they are supplying; for taking off, for during the flight and for the landing.

Once you learn how to get rid of your flying fear you will relish your new transformation and you will see a better you; you will convert moments of anxiety into moments of tranquility during you journey among all the other benefits that arises from learning how to meditate. You will be enriched by the self discovery and the control you are going to have in other areas of your life.

# Meditation - Know About Transcendental Meditation

True, the word meditation immediately brings to mind the picture of an old sage, with a flowing white beard and a head full of silky white hair contemplating on issues that mostly concern the spiritual side of life. It does sound very mystical and intimidating however it is not a pre-requisite to practicing meditation.

However Maharishi Mahesh Yogi, founder of the transcendental meditation does sport a similar look and while his habit of giggling during interviews, may have earned him the nickname "giggling guru" he does have a bunch of dedicated followers.

## What is Transcendental meditation?

Transcendental meditation is said to be a set of Hindu meditation techniques, involving the chanting of a mantra which is basically just the name of a Hindu god. However, transcendental meditation, according to its leaders and followers, requires just two 20 minutes a day spent in a state they call restful alertness.

According to them, it doesn't need you to concentrate or focus on anything. And it supposedly works even without you believing that it does. The followers of transcendental meditation also say that at the height of restful awareness, the mind transcends all mental actions which they term as Transcendental Consciousness. They further claim that scientific studies have proven that experiencing this state of the mind brings about higher IQ, creativity, learning, moral reasoning, and even a better neurological functioning of one's body. In short, transcendental meditation frees the mind and body of their inhibitions and releases all the suppressed natural capabilities vital to leading a happy life.

Because of the methods and techniques involved in practicing transcendental meditation it can rather easily be mistook for a religion or a cult. Another contributing reason why it may be mistook for a religion or cult is because it is often referred to as the "Science of Creative Intelligence", which incidentally is now a degree at the Maharishi University of Management in Fairfield, Iowa.

The university also boasts of "a Full Range of Academic Disciplines for Successful Management of All Fields of Life". The group of people opposing transcendental meditation's claims also point out that several health and beauty products are being sold on the university premises for people who want to "improve" their body as much as their mind.

However the most unbelievable claim of all claims surrounding transcendental meditation is that practicing it enables its followers to fly - or levitate. This was probably disproved because they do not insist on being able to fly anymore, though some others still declare to have possessed supernatural and paranormal capabilities like becoming invisible. Along with flying, this claim too remains unproven to this date.

A former transcendental follower once said that most meditation methods are quite similar to the transcendental meditation, the only difference being that the latter is wrapped up in questionable publicity claims and stunts. The best way to practice transcendental meditation is to follow the techniques and practices for the sole purpose of relaxing the mind and body and not get swayed by it's dubious claims.

The Transcendental Meditation technique may be an effective and safe non-pharmaceutical aid for treating ADHD, according to a promising new study published this month in the peer-reviewed online journal Current Issues in Education.

The pilot study followed a group of middle school students with ADHD who were meditating twice a day in school. After three months, researchers found over 50 percent reduction in stress and anxiety and improvements in ADHD symptoms.

**Effect exceeds expectations**

"The effect was much greater than we expected," said Sarina J. Grosswald, Ed.D., a George Washington University-trained cognitive learning specialist and lead researcher on the study. "The children also showed improvements in attention, working memory, organization, and behavior regulation."

Grosswald said that after the in-school meditation routine began, "teachers reported they were able to teach more, and students were able to learn more because they were less stressed and anxious."

## Stress interferes with the ability to learn

Prior research shows ADHD children have slower brain development and a reduced ability to cope with stress. "Stress interferes with the ability to learn-it shuts down the brain," said William Stixrud, Ph.D., a Silver Spring, Maryland, clinical neuropsychologist and co-author of the study.

"Medication for ADHD is very effective for some children, but it is marginally or not effective for others. Even for those children who show improved symptoms with the medication, the improvement is often insufficient or accompanied by troubling side effects," Stixrud said. "Virtually everyone finds it difficult to pay attention, organize themselves and get things done when they're under stress. So it stands to reason that the TM technique which reduces stress and organizes brain function would reduce ADHD symptoms."

While in some cases a child cannot function without medication, there is growing concern about the health risks and side effects associated with the common ADHD medications, including mood swings, insomnia, tics, slowed growth, and heart problems. In 2006 the FDA required manufacturers to place warning labels on ADHD medications, listing the potential serious health risks.

These high risks and growing concerns are fueling parents' search for alternatives that may be safer for their kids.

The study was conducted in a private K-12 school for children with language-based learning disabilities. Participation was restricted to 10 students, ages 11-14, who had pre-existing diagnoses of ADHD. About half of the students were on medication. The students meditated at school in a group for 10 minutes, morning and afternoon.

To determine the influence of the TM technique, at the beginning and end of the three-month period, parents, teachers and students completed standard ADHD assessment inventories measuring stress and anxiety, behavior and social competency, and executive function. Students were also given a battery of performance tests to measure cognitive functioning.

"The results were quite remarkable"

Andy and Daryl Schoenbach's daughter was diagnosed with ADHD in second grade. Like most ADHD children she was taking medication. "The medication helped but had mixed results-she still lost focus, had meltdowns, and the medications affected her sleep and appetite," said Andy, who lives with Daryl in Washington D.C. "She was not performing close to her potential and we didn't see the situation improving. So at the end of seventh grade when her doctor recommended increasing the medication, we decided it was time to take a different course-stopping the medication and using Transcendental Meditation."

"The results were quite remarkable," Daryl said. "The twice daily meditations smoothed things out, gave her perspective, and enabled her to be in greater control of her own life when things started falling apart. It took some time, but it gradually changed the way she handled crises and enabled her to feel confident that she could take on greater challenges -in her own words, 'climb a mountain.'"

"Everyone noticed the change," Andy added.

Grosswald explained that there is substantial research showing the effectiveness of the TM technique for reducing stress and anxiety, and improving cognitive functioning among the general population.

"What's significant about these new findings is that among children who have difficulty with focus and attention, we see the same results. TM doesn't require concentration, controlling the mind or disciplined focus. The fact that these children are able to do TM, and do it easily shows us that this technique may be particularly well suited for children with ADHD," she said.

This study was funded by the Abramson Family Foundation and the Institute for Community Enrichment.

A second, recently completed TM-ADHD study with a control group measured brain function using electroencephalography (EEG). Preliminary data shows that three months practice of the technique resulted in significant positive changes in brain functioning during visual-motor skills. Changes were specifically seen in the circuitry of the brain associated with attention and distractibility. After six months TM practice, measurements of distractibility moved into the normal range.

A third, $2 million TM-ADHD study, to be funded in part by a grant from The David Lynch Foundation, will more fully investigate the effects of the technique on ADHD and other learning disorders.

**Facts about ADHD**

Attention Deficit Hyperactivity Disorder (ADHD)

- ✓ The Center for Disease Control reports that nearly 50 percent of the 4.5 million children (ages 4-17) in the United States diagnosed with ADHD are on ADHD medication-and the majority of those on medication stay on it in adulthood.
- ✓ The rate of prescriptions for Attention Deficit Hyperactivity Disorder in the U.S. has increasing by a factor of five since 1991-with production of ADHD medicines up 2,000 percent in 9 years.
- ✓ The commonly used drugs for ADHD are stimulants (amphetamines). These drugs can cause persistent and negative side effects, including sleep disturbances, reduced appetite, weight loss, suppressed growth, and mood disorders. The side effects are frequently treated with

additional medications to manage insomnia or mood swings. Almost none of the medications prescribed for insomnia or mood disturbances are approved by the Food and Drug Administration (FDA) for use with children.

✓ The long-term health effects of ADHD medications are not fully known, but evidence suggests risks of cardiac disorders and sudden death, liver damage and psychiatric events. It has also been found that children on long-term medication have significantly higher rates of delinquency, substance use, and stunted physical growth.

# The Holosync Solution to Learning Meditation

Holosync is a meditation course that uses break-through technology to create deep states of meditation. It works on the scientific discovery that you can slow down your brainwaves by listening to specific sound frequencies. These frequencies are recorded in a special way that causes your brain to produce the same slow rhythmic brainwaves that are produced during Zen Meditation.

Meditation and mastering your brainwaves is the key to realizing your dreams, ambitions and achieving your goals in life. Mastering your brain and your brainwaves gives you the power to become master over your entire life!

Traditionally the only way to slow down your brainwaves was through meditation. There have been many studies and much research conducted into the benefits of meditation. People who regularly practise meditation are healthier, more emotionally balanced, less stressed and to a greater or lesser degree they are happier.

After many years of practise it is possible to meditate and program your brain with your specific goals. Re-programming the subconscious mind in this way can have dramatic positive effects on your life.

Those dedicated individuals, who have devoted years to the quest, can easily lower their brainwaves so they can program their mind with any goal they choose. Many studies and a lot of research data supports the belief that using visualization and/or affirmations as part of goal-setting dramatically increases your chances of achieving that goal.

Fortunately though, you do not need to learn meditation or spend years perfecting it anymore. With Holosync you can, within a few short minutes, enter into deep meditative states and start to reap the rewards. This means Holosync can give you all the benefits of meditation without the years of effort learning how to do it!

If Holosync is used daily, as prescribed, the health, mental and physical benefits you receive will be identical to those you would receive if you learned how to meditate the traditional way. However, Holosync gets results much quicker.

If you were to learn meditation it may take you many years to perfect the deeper states. Knowing how to enter these deeper states, where you dramatically lower your brainwave frequenies, can take a life-time to learn. However, with Holosync you enter these states on the very first listening.

Holosync eliminates the need to spend hours a day, over the span of decades, learning how to meditate deeply. Holosync instantly provides the necessary stimuli to create the specific brainwaves needed to enter deep meditative states.

Some of the benefits of Holosync, that users have reported, include:

- ✓ Deep meditation.
- ✓ Deep relaxation.
- ✓ Increased calmness.
- ✓ Decreased Stress.
- ✓ More Creativity.
- ✓ Increased Focus.
- ✓ Better Problem Solving.
- ✓ Better Retention of Learned Information.
- ✓ And More Confidence
- ✓ 10.And many more.

However, Holosync does not just slow down your brainwaves or produce specific brainwave frequencies. Although this, in itself, is highly beneficial to your health there is another positive by-product of using holosync which is extremely important.

Using Holosync you will align both hemispheres of your brain to create whole-brain synchronization. Both hemispheres of the brain become aligned, harmonious and function as one unit. This is important as, normally, either the right or the left hemisphere of the brain is dominant over the other. To simplify this we can say you are either more creative or more analytical. With whole-brain functionality, created by Holosync, you can unleash the side of you that has been dormant.

An added avantage of using Holosync means that both your creative side and your analytical side are active at the same time. You can tap into your intuition while also being able to make practical analytical decisions.

The whole-brain functioning produced by Holosync also makes you much more productive as both hemispheres of your brain work together in harmony. The same positive effects are evident in people who have regularly practised meditation for many years. However with Holosync you can do it in a fraction of the time.

The power behind the Holosync recordings is binaural beats. However unlike other recordings that use this technology, Holosync uses binaural beats in a very specific way to deliberately entrain the brain through a series of deepening audios that gradually entrain the brain to its highest functionality - something that is not currently offered by another brain entrainment program.

This means that sustained use of Holosync means you retain all the benefits of its use for life! Now as I previously mentioned you can get the same results from practising meditation but, if you are like the average person, the time it takes to learn this ancient art is in years if not decades. Holosync does it instantly.

CPSIA information can be obtained
at www.ICGtesting.com
Printed in the USA
LVHW082011040521
686472LV00002B/228